Delicious and Healthy Vegetarian Recipes

Eat Vegetarion As Good As Meat

Copyright © 2021

DEDICATION

Contents

Maple Mustard Tempeh Meal Prep Bowls

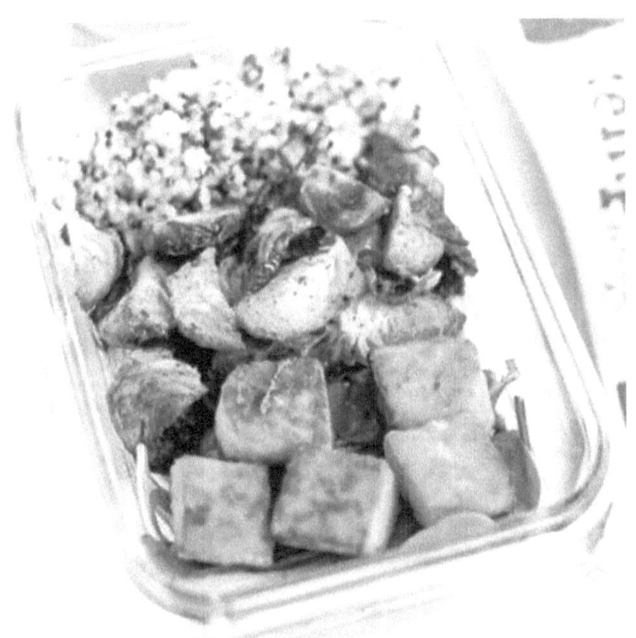

Prep Time: 2 hours 15 minutes

Cook Time: 40 minutes

Total Time: 2 hours 55 minutes

Yield: 4 bowls

INGREDIENTS

- 8 oz package Original or Three-Grain Lightlife tempeh, chopped into 20 cubes

- 2 lbs brussels sprouts, trimmed and halved or quartered

- 2–3 Tablespoons olive oil + 1–2 teaspoons

- 1 teaspoon sea salt

- 1 teaspoon pepper

- 1 cup dry quinoa

- 3 cups mixed greens

MAPLE MUSTARD MARINADE/DRESSING

- 1 lemon, juiced

- 1 Tablespoon apple cider vinegar

- 2 Tablespoons maple syrup

- 2 Tablespoons dijon mustard

- 1/2 teaspoon minced garlic

- 1/4 teaspoon sea salt

- ground pepper, to taste

- 1/4 cup olive oil

INSTRUCTIONS

1. Make marinade by whisking together all of the ingredients in a large bowl or container. Place tempeh cubes into the bowl and place in the fridge to marinade for at least 2 hours, preferably overnight.

2. Roast brussels sprouts: Preheat oven to 400°F. Wash, trim and chop brussels sprouts before adding them to a roasting pan with olive oil, sea salt and pepper. Toss to combine and roast for 35-40 minutes, or until cooked through with some golden brown spots. Be sure to toss around the 20-minute mark.

3. While brussels sprouts are roasting, cook quinoa by adding 1 cup dry quinoa to 2 cups of water or broth in a saucepan. Bring liquid to a boil, reduce heat to a simmer, cover and cook for 15 minutes, or until no liquid remains. Remove from heat and use a fork to fluff the quinoa.

4. Cook tempeh by adding 1-2 teaspoons of oil to a pan over medium heat. Use a slotted spoon to remove tempeh from the marinade and place in the pan. Cook tempeh cubes until all sides are golden brown, about 6-8 minutes. Remove from heat.

5. At this point, you can serve the dish as is or let everything cool before dividing everything into four meal prep containers. For the containers, each gets 3/4 cup of cooked quinoa, about 1 1/2 cups roasted brussels sprouts, 5 cubes of tempeh and 3/4 cup mixed greens. Place leftover marinade in a storage container and save to use as a dressing for the bowls when ready to serve.

NUTRITION

Per serving: 553 calories, 29 g fat (4 g saturated), 56 g carbs, 13 g sugar, 188 mg sodium, 16 g fiber, 23 g protein

Mediterranean Farro Salad

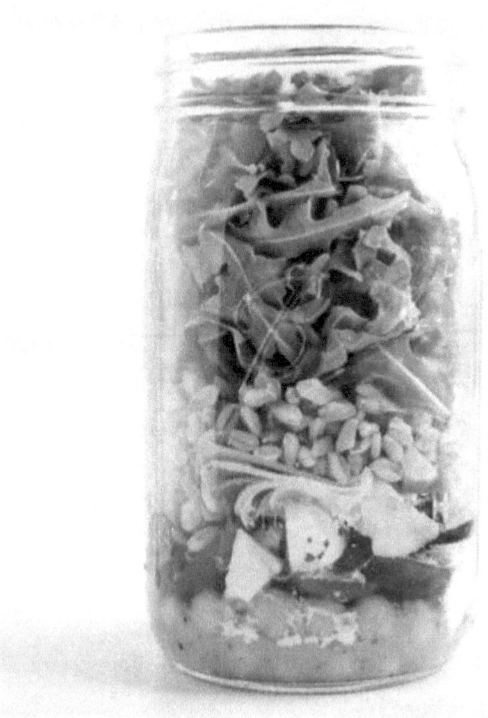

Prep Time: 10 minutes

Cook Time: 30 minutes

Total Time: 40 minutes

Yield: 1

INGREDIENTS

- ½ cup cooked chickpeas

- ¼ cup chopped tomatoes

- ¼ cup marinated artichoke hearts

- ¼ cup olives, chopped

- 2–3 mozzarella balls, chopped

- ½ cup cooked farro

- 2 cups arugula

- 1 Tablespoon chopped sun-dried tomatoes

RED WINE VINAIGRETTE (MAKES 3/4 CUP)

- 1/3 cup red wine vinegar

- 1 Tablespoon Dijon mustard

- 1–2 cloves garlic, minced

- 1 teaspoon maple syrup or honey

- 3/4 teaspoon sea salt

- 1/2 teaspoon black pepper

- 1/2 cup extra virgin olive oil

INSTRUCTIONS

1. Make the dressing by whisking together all the ingredients in a small bowl or glass jar.

2. If it isn't pre-cooked, cook your farro according to package directions

3. For a mason jar: Add 2-3 Tablespoons of dressing into a large, wide-mouth mason jar, then start layering ingredients in this order: chickpeas, tomatoes, mozzarella balls, olives, artichoke hearts, farro, arugula, sundried tomatoes.

4. For a meal prep container: Line bottom of container with arugula and layer all ingredients in columns/sections on top. Store dressing in a separate container.

NUTRITION

Per serving: 667 calories, 35 g fat, g carbs, 64 g sugar, 11 g fiber, 24 g protein

Vegan Mediterranean Bowls

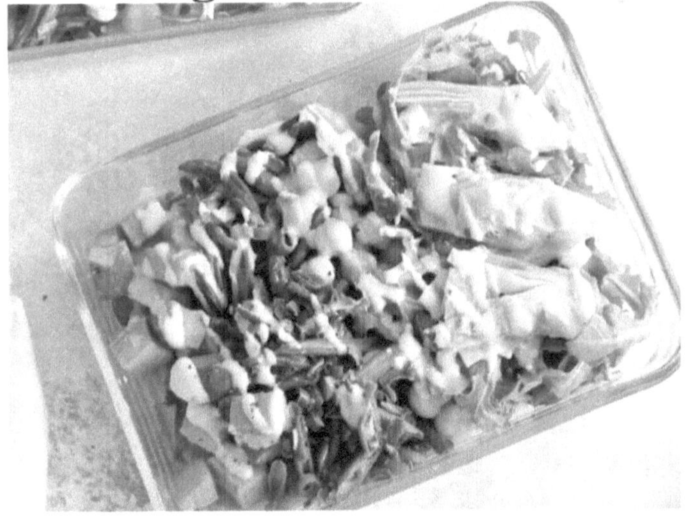

Prep Time: 15 mins
Cook Time: 35 mins
Total Time: 50 mins
Yield: 4

INGREDIENTS

For the roasted veggies:

- 2 large sweet potatoes, diced
- 16oz fresh or frozen green beans, trimmed*
- 1 1/2 tbsp oil of choice, divided
- 1 tsp kosher salt, divided

For the lemon tahini sauce:

- 1/4 cup tahini
- 2 tbsp lemon juice
- 2 tbsp water
- 1/2 tsp garlic powder
- 1/4 tsp kosher salt
- Freshly ground black epper

For assembly:

- 1–6oz jar marinated artichoke hearts in oil, chopped
- 1–15oz can chickpeas
- 3 cups arugula

- 1 avocado, diced (optional)

INSTRUCTIONS

1. Preheat oven to 425F and line two baking sheets with parchment paper. Toss potatoes, 3/4 tbsp oil, and 1/2 tsp salt in a bowl. Spread onto baking sheet. In the same bowl, toss green beans, remaining 3/4 tbsp oil, 1/2 tsp salt in bowl. Spread on other baking sheet. Place both sheets in oven and bake for 35-40 minutes, tossing halfway through.

2. Meanwhile, combine tahini, lemon juice, garlic powder, salt, and pepper in a small bowl. Stir in water until smooth, adding another tablespoon if needed.

3. In 4 3-cup rectangular glass Pyrex containers (or containers of choice), evenly distribute 3-4 artichokes, 1/3 cup chickpeas, a handful of arugula, 3/4 cup roasted sweet potatoes, and 1/2 cup roasted green beans. Serve drizzled evenly with lemon tahini sauce. Add avocado right before serving or add the night before with a squeeze of lemon juice.

NUTRITION

Per serving: 657 calories, 35 g fat, 64 g carbs, 7 g sugar, 11 g fiber, 24 g protein

No-Bake PB & J Energy Bites

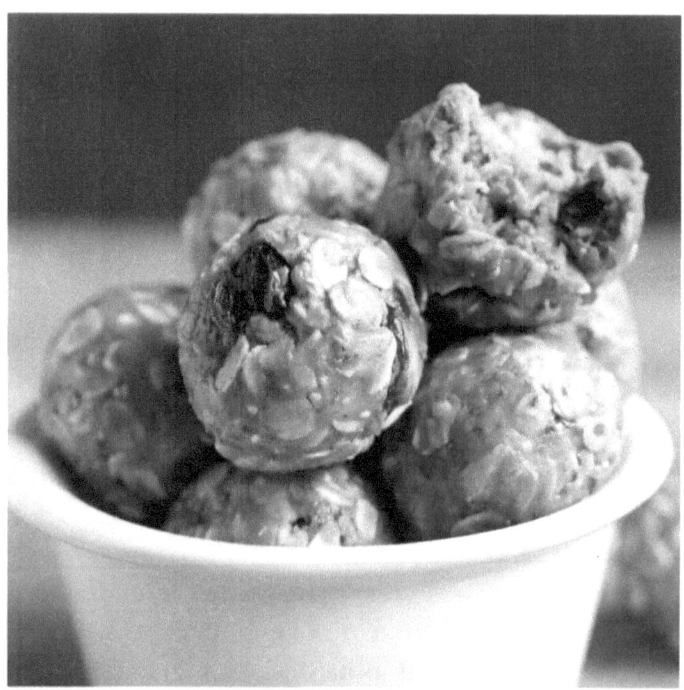

Prep Time: 15 mins
Total Time: 15 mins
Yield: 14 bites

INGREDIENTS

- 1/2 cup creamy salted peanut butter (or almond, cashew, or sunbutter)
- 1/4 cup maple syrup (or sub finely chopped dates)
- 2 Tbsp vegan protein powder* (optional - just omit if you don't have any)

- 1 1/4 cup gluten-free rolled oats*
- 2 1/2 Tbsp flaxseed meal
- 2 Tbsp chia seeds
- 1/4 cup dried fruit (i.e. dried strawberries, cherries, blueberries, cranberries)

INSTRUCTIONS

1. To a large mixing bowl, add peanut butter, maple syrup, protein powder, rolled oats, flaxseed meal, chia seeds, and dried fruit of choice. Mix until well combined. If too dry/crumbly, add more peanut butter or maple syrup. If too sticky or wet, add a little bit more oats or flaxseed meal.
2. Chill in the refrigerator for 5 minutes. Then scoop out 1 1/2 Tbsp amounts (I like using **this scoop**) and roll into balls. The "dough" should yield about 13-14 balls (amount as original recipe is written // adjust if altering batch size).
3. Enjoy immediately and store well-sealed leftovers in the refrigerator for 1 week or in the freezer up to 1 month (or more).

NUTRITION

Per serving: 125 calories, 1.1 g fat, 13.8 g carbs, 5.9 g sugar, 45 mg sodium, 1.8 g fiber, 4.4 g protein

Peanut Butter Overnight Oats

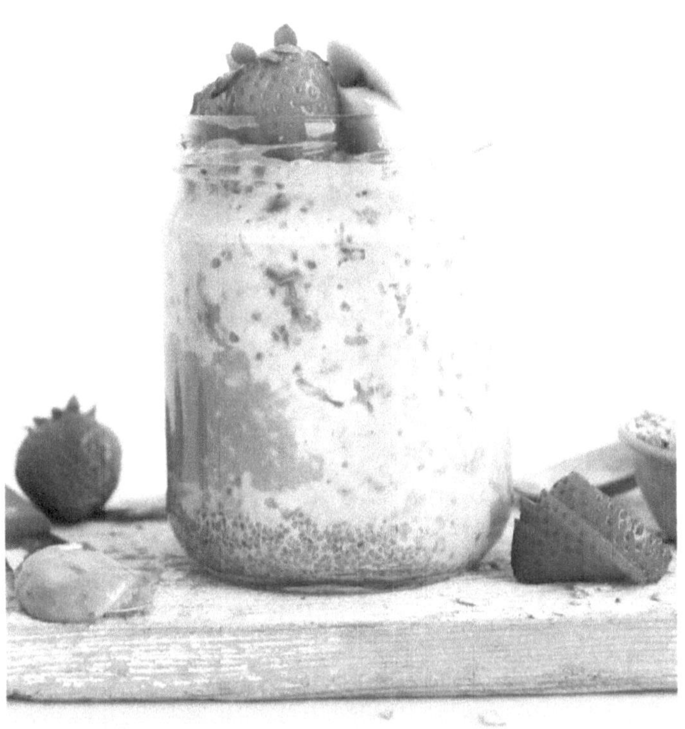

Prep Time: 6 hours 5 minutes
Total Time: 6 hours 5 minutes

Yield: 1

INGREDIENTS

OATS

- 1/2 cup unsweetened plain almond milk (or sub other dairy-free milks, such as coconut, soy, or hemp!)
- 3/4 Tbsp chia seeds
- 2 Tbsp natural salted peanut butter or almond butter (creamy or crunchy // or sub other nut or seed butter)
- 1 Tbsp maple syrup (or sub coconut sugar, organic brown sugar, or stevia to taste)
- 1/2 cup gluten-free rolled oats (rolled oats are best, vs. steel cut or quick cooking)

TOPPINGS optional

- Sliced banana, strawberries, or raspberries
- Flaxseed meal or additional chia seed
- Granola

INSTRUCTIONS

1. To a mason jar or small bowl with a lid, add almond milk, chia seeds, peanut butter, and maple syrup (or other sweetener) and stir with a spoon to combine. The peanut butter doesn't need to be completely mixed with the almond milk (doing so leaves swirls of peanut butter to enjoy the next day).
2. Add oats and stir a few more times. Then press down with a spoon to ensure all oats have been moistened and are immersed in almond milk.
3. Cover securely with a lid or seal and set in the refrigerator overnight (or for at least 6 hours) to set/soak.

4. The next day, open and enjoy as is or garnish with desired toppings (see options above). See more flavor/topping suggestions in the blog post above!

OPTIONAL: You can also heat your oats in the microwave for 45-60 seconds (just ensure there's enough room at the top of your jar to allow for expansion and prevent overflow), or transfer oats to a saucepan and heat over medium heat until warmed through. Add more liquid as needed if oats get too thick/dry.

5. Overnight oats will keep in the refrigerator for 2-3 days, though best within the first 12-24 hours in our experience. Not freezer friendly.

NUTRITION

Per serving: 454 calories, 23.9 g fat (2 g saturated), 50.9 g carbs, 14.9 g sugar, 162 mg sodium, 12 g fiber, 14.6 g protein

Sweet Potato Black Bean Enchiladas

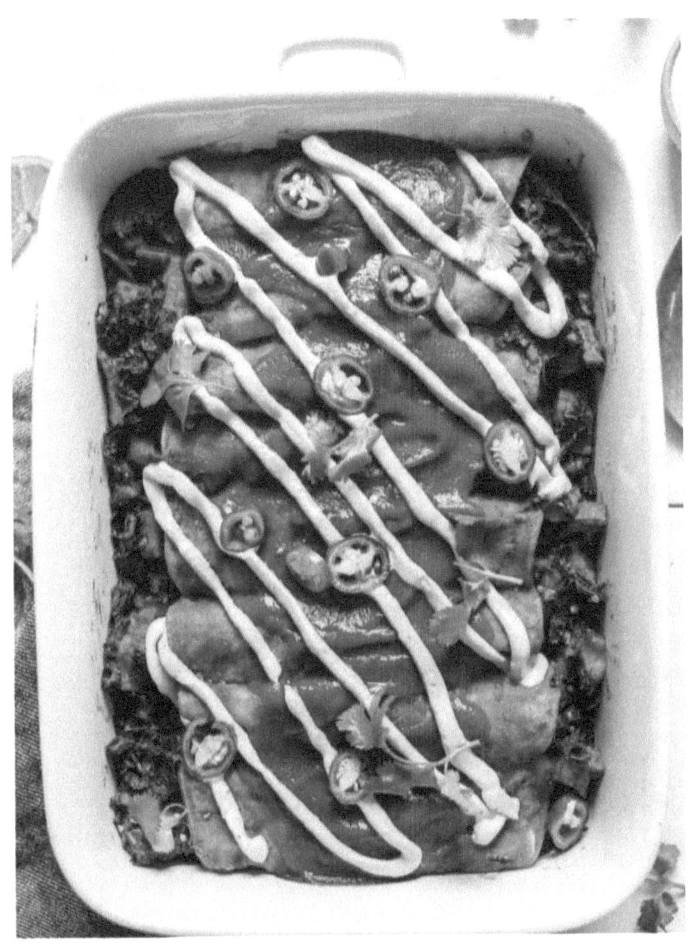

Prep Time: 15 minutes
Cook Time: 40 minutes
Total Time: 55 minutes

Yield: 10 (enchiladas)

INGREDIENTS

TORTILLAS

- 10 small yellow or white corn tortillas*

FILLING

- 3 cups cubed sweet potatoes (skin on)
- 1 Tbsp coconut or avocado oil (or sub water)
- 1 tsp ground cumin
- 1/2 tsp smoked paprika
- 1/4 tsp sea salt
- 2 cups chopped kale (or other sturdy green)
- 2 Tbsp (30 ml) water
- 1 15-ounce can black beans* (drained // or sub pinto or refried beans)
- 1/4 cup Red Enchilada Sauce (or store-bought)

SAUCE

- 3 cups Red Enchilada Sauce (divided // or store-bought)

FOR SERVING optional

- Cilantro
- Guacamole, avocado, or Avocado Crema (see notes for recipe)

INSTRUCTIONS

1. Preheat oven to 400 degrees F (204 C) and position a rack in the middle of the oven.

2. Add cubed sweet potato to one large baking sheet (or more as needed) and drizzle with oil (or water), cumin, paprika, and salt. Toss to combine.

3. Bake for 20-25 minutes or until sweet potatoes are fork tender and slightly caramelized. Set aside to cool. Also reduce oven heat to 350 degrees F (176 C).

4. In the meantime, add your kale to a large cast-iron or metal skillet over medium heat with 2 Tbsp (30 ml) water. Cover and steam for about 4-5 minutes or until kale is slightly softened but still vibrant green. Uncover and set aside. (You could also sauté the kale in a bit of oil if you prefer.)

5. Add drained black beans to a mixing bowl with steamed kale and roasted sweet potatoes. Add the smaller measurement of enchilada sauce to the kale and sweet potatoes and stir to combine.

6. Wrap tortillas in damp cloth towel and microwave to warm for 30 seconds to make more pliable. (Alternatively, place wrapped tortillas directly on oven rack for a few minutes to heat through.) This will help them become more pliable and easy to roll.

7. Pour about one third of the enchilada sauce into the bottom of a 9x13-inch (3 quart | or similar shaped) baking dish. Spread to coat.

8. Lay one corn tortilla down in the saucy dish to coat. Then flip it over to coat the other side. Fill with ~1/3 cup of the filling. Then roll up and lay seam-side down at the edge of the dish. Continue until all tortillas are filled and rolled, adding more sauce as needed to moisten tortillas. Add any remaining filling to the edges of the dish. If you run out of space to roll the tortillas in the baking dish, continue saucing, filling, and rolling them on a small serving plate.

9. Pour remaining enchilada sauce over the top of the enchiladas in a stripe down the middle. TIP: Use less sauce for slightly drier enchiladas. The more sauce you use, the more tender the tortillas will become.

10. Bake at 350 degrees F (176C) for 15-20 minutes or until warmed through. Top with desired toppings and serve. We went with

fresh jalapeño, cilantro, and avocado crema (recipe below), but these enchiladas are delicious on their own!

11.   Leftovers will keep covered in the refrigerator up to 3 days or in the freezer up to 1 month, though best when fresh. Reheat in a 350-degree F (176 C) oven for 15-20 minutes or until warmed through.

NUTRITION

Per serving: 230.4 calories, 2.9 g fat (1.3 g saturated), 45.1 g carbs, 6.9 g sugar, 480 mg sodium, 10/4 g fiber, 7.4 g protein

Freezable Veggie Burger

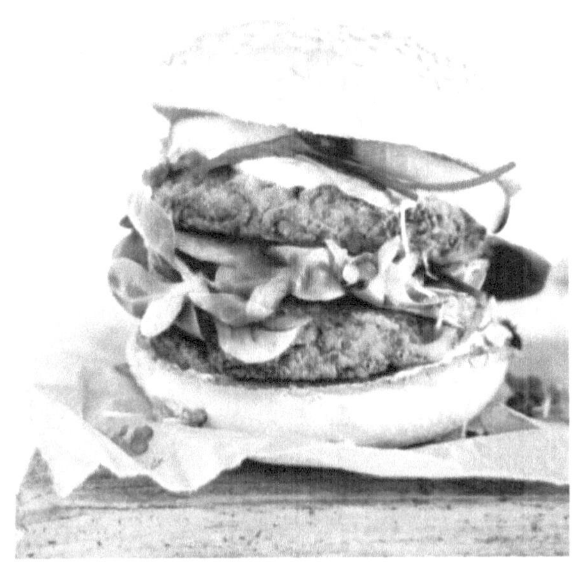

Prep Time: 25 min

Cook Time: 25 min

Total Time: 50 minutes

Yield: 5-7

INGREDIENTS

- 1 cup cooked, drained chickpeas beans (or navy beans)

- 1 cup chopped mixed vegetables (I used carrot, cauliflower, and broccoli)

- 1/4 cup red onion, diced

- 1/2 cup sunflower seeds

- 1 Tbsp pine nuts or pumpkin seed

- 1/2 tsp dried herbs or 2 tbsp fresh dill (i.e dill, oregano, etc.)

- 1/4 cup fresh basil leaves

- 2 tsp ground flaxseed seed

- 1 Tbsp tamari sauce or coconut aminos for soy free option

- 1 tsp minced garlic

- 1/4 tsp kosher salt

- Optional spices – dash paprika, red pepper, or cayenne (to taste)

- 1/4 cup gluten free flour (cassava flour, arrowroot, potato flour, or 1:1 GF all work). You can also use around 3 tbsp coconut flour.

INSTRUCTIONS

1. Preheat oven to 375F.

2. Place everything except the flour in a food processor or blender and blend until almost smooth. You can leave it a little chunky so that vegetable pieces still remain visible.

3. Next, add in a little of your flour (1/4 cup gluten free flour) and pulse gently to mix. If the batter is too thin, add a little more flour. You want to make sure the batter can hold together. Form batter into a ball, wrap in plastic and let it chill in fridge for 20 minutes. This is optional, but it helps hold better before baking.

4. Next, oil a baking sheet or line with parchment paper.

5. Shape the veggie/nut mixture into 5-7 burger patties, about 1/2 inch thickness and width of the palm of your hand. Flatten and place on the baking sheet. The burgers will not expand so you can line them up close.

6. Bake about 15 minutes on one side, then GENTLY take a spatula and flip them to the other side.

7. Bake again another 10-12 minutes or so. Burgers will be a little golden brown and slightly crispy on the edges when they are finished.

8. Feel free to freeze them in foil or wax paper, but let them cool first before doing so. You may also freeze the uncooked burgers between wax paper to keep/store before cooking.

NUTRITION

Per serving: 195 calories, 13 g fat (1.8 g saturated), 15.4 g carbs, 1.6 g sugar, 465.6 mg sodium, 6.6 g fiber, 7.4 g proteinPer serving: 657 calories, 35 g fat, 64 g carbs, 7 g sugar, 11 g fiber, 24 g protein

Strawberry Protein Muffins

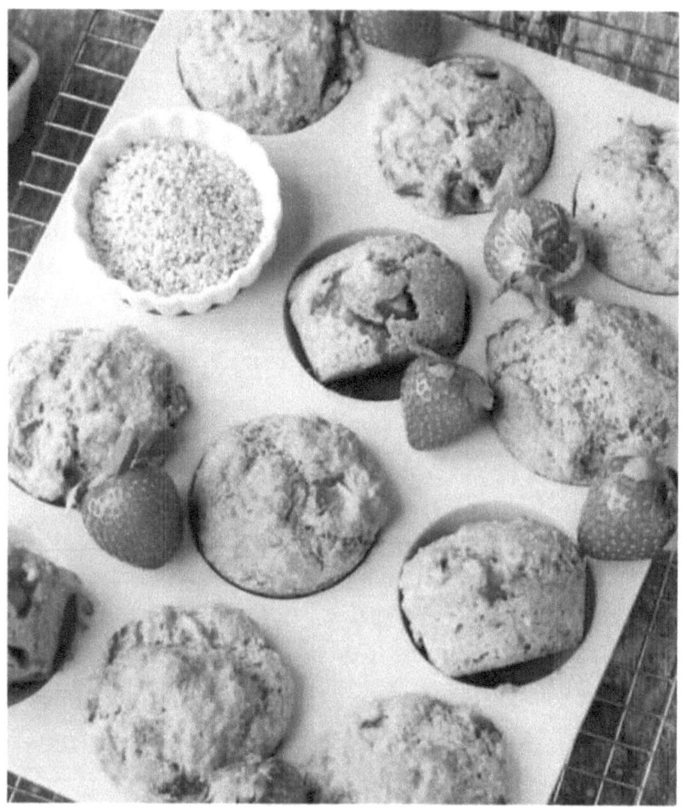

Prep Time: 15 mins

Cook Time: 25 mins

Total Time: 40 mins

Yield: 6 muffins

INGREDIENTS

- 2 tablespoons ground chia seeds or chia seeds (divided)
- 5 tablespoons dairy-free butter
- ½ cup coconut sugar
- ½ cup plus 2 tablespoons dairy-free milk
- 1 tablespoon lemon juice
- 1½ cups whole wheat flour
- 1½ teaspoons baking powder
- ½ teaspoon baking soda
- ¼ teaspoon salt
- ¼ cup raw shelled hempseed
- ½ cup strawberries (chopped)

INSTRUCTIONS

1. Preheat the oven to 375°F.
2. Grease the inside of a six-cup muffin tin and set aside.
3. Mix 1 tablespoon ground chia seeds together with 3 tablespoons water and set aside.
4. Using an electric mixer, beat together the butter and sugar in a large bowl until light and fluffy, about 3 minutes. Add the chia seed mixture and mix again. Add the milk and lemon juice. Mix well.
5. Add the flour, baking powder, baking soda, salt, hempseed, and the remaining tablespoon ground chia seeds to a medium bowl. Mix. Add the flour mixture to the wet mixture and beat until just combined. It will be a sticky batter.
6. Fold in the strawberries.
7. Divide the batter between the muffin cups. Fill at least three-quarters full.
8. Bake for 25 minutes or until a toothpick inserted into the center comes out clean.

NUTRITION

Per serving: 295 calories, 15 g fat (3 g saturated), 40 g carbs, 17 g sugar, 243 mg sodium, 4 g fiber, 8 g protein

Greek Cauliflower Salad Bowls

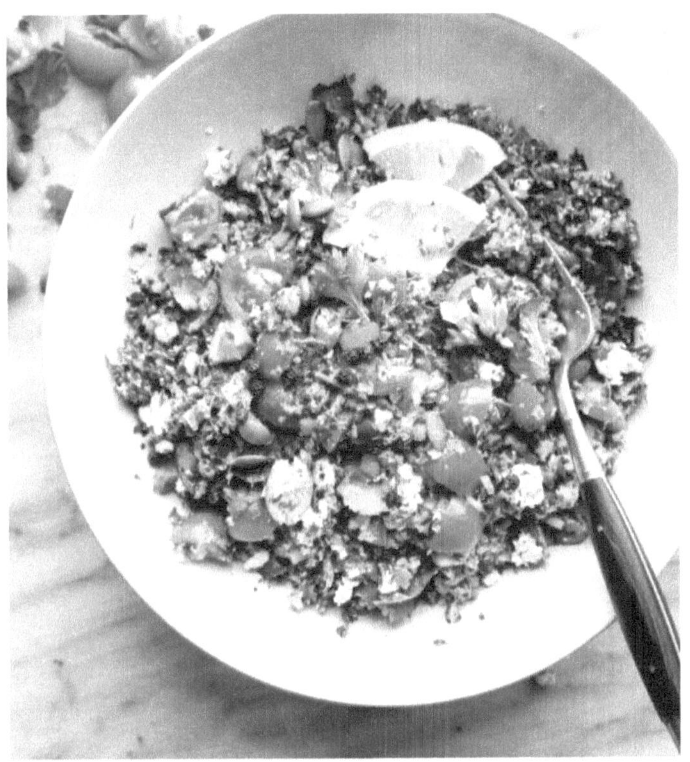

Prep Time: 15

Total Time: 15

Yield: 3

INGREDIENTS

• 1 small to medium head cauliflower (riced) – if you prefer to buy premade cauliflower rice, use 3 to 4 cups riced.

• 1–2 tbsp of olive oil (2 tbsp if using a large amount of cauliflower)

- 1/2 teaspoon minced garlic (or 1/4 tsp garlic powder)

- 1/2 teaspoon fine sea salt

- 1/2 teaspoon ground black pepper

- 1/4 cup pumpkin seeds

- 1 cup grape leaves – Found in grocery aisle – a jar or can (shredded and pressed clean to remove extra water).

- 1 cup cherry tomatoes – diced/sliced

- 1/4 cup chopped fresh basil, parsley, or cilantro!

- 5–7 marinated green olives (or regular stuffed olives)

- 1/2 lemon, juiced

- 1 ounce or more crumbled goat cheese (soft) – skip for dairy free/vegan option! Or see notes for alternatives

INSTRUCTIONS

1. Remove the stem from the cauliflower and cut the cauliflower head into four or five sections. Place one or two sections of the cauliflower, depending on size, into a food processor and pulse until cauliflower rice is formed, usually 3 or 4 pulses.

2. Repeat for each section of the cauliflower.

3. Place the cauliflower rice in a large bowl. Add 1-2 tbsp olive oil, garlic, salt, pepper and pumpkin seeds, and toss to combine.

4. For a fresh cauliflower salad, mix the cauliflower rice with the chopped grape leaves (preparation instructions below) and tomatoes. Alternatively you can lightly toast the cauliflower rice on an

oiled baking sheet, spread out evenly. Bake for 10-15 minutes at 375F, tossing once during baking. Remove and let cool.

5. To prepare the grape leaves, rinse the grape leaves with water to remove the excess salt. Press the grape leaves with a paper towel to remove the excess water. Chop or shred grape leaves and set aside.

6. Dice the tomatoes, herbs, and olives to your liking. Place in s large bowl with the cauliflower rice, and then add the grape leaves. Toss together, mixing well. Add a fresh squeeze of lemon, salt and pepper to taste, and red pepper flakes.

7. GARNISH with a hefty dose of crumbled goat cheese, Red pepper flakes, herbs (cilantro or basil), and lemon slices.

8. You can serve straight from one large bowl or serve into 2 -3 smaller bowls!

NUTRITION

Per serving: 232 calories, 17.7 g fat (3.9 g saturated), 14.2 g carbs, 4.2 g sugar, 609.1 mg sodium, 5.9 g fiber, 9.4 g protein

Beet Power Salad

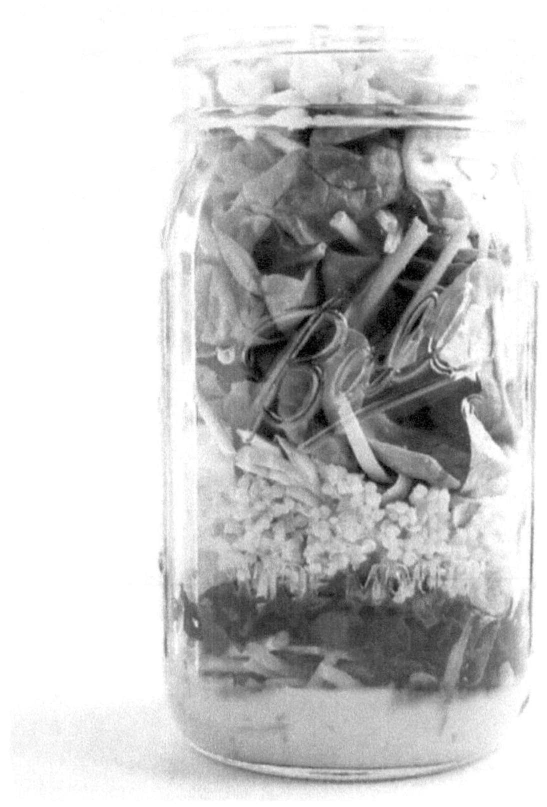

rep Time: 10 minutes

otal Time: 10 minutes

ield: 1

NGREDIENTS

- 2 cooked beets, chopped or shredded

- ¼ cup shredded carrots

- ½ cup cooked quinoa
- ¼ cup shredded brussels sprouts
- 2 cups leafy greens (I like baby spinach)
- 2 Tablespoons golden raisins
- 2 Tablespoons goat cheese crumbles
- 1 Tablespoon cashews

Zesty Tahini Dressing

- 1/4 cup tahini
- 1/4 cup apple cider vinegar
- 1/4 cup lemon juice
- 1/4 cup low-sodium tamari or soy sauce
- 1/2 cup nutritional yeast
- 1 Tablespoon minced garlic

INSTRUCTIONS

1. If your vegetables aren't chopped or shredded already, prep them!

2. Make the dressing by whisking together all the ingredients in a small bowl or glass jar.

3. For a mason jar: Add 2-3 Tablespoons of dressing into a large, wide-mouth mason jar, then start layering ingredients in this order: carrots, beets, raisins, quinoa, brussels sprouts, leafy greens, goat cheese crumbles, cashews.

4. For a meal prep container: Line bottom of container with leafy greens and layer all ingredients in columns/sections on top. Store dressing in a separate container.

NUTRITION

Per serving: 379 calories, 14 g fat, 49 g carbs, 14 g sugar, 12 g fiber, 19 g protein

Vegan Sweet Potato Buddha Bowl

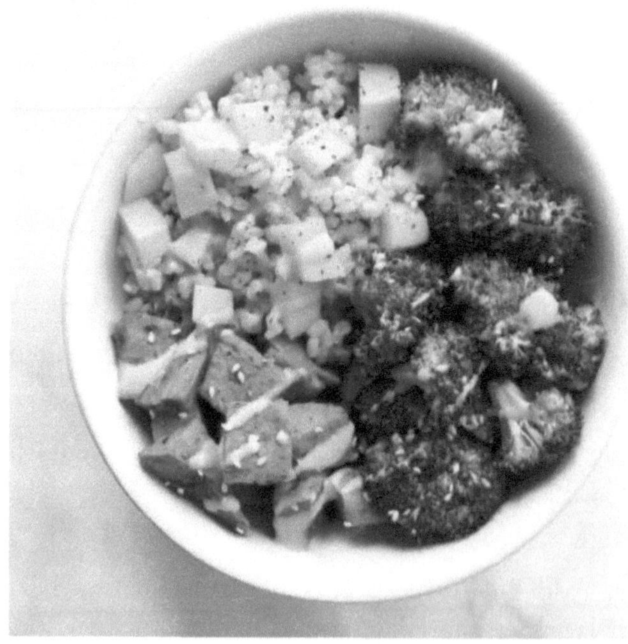

Prep Time: 15 minutes
Cook Time: 45 minutes

Total Time: 1 hour

Yield: 4

INGREDIENTS

For the roasted veggies:

- 1 large head of broccoli, cut into florets

- 2 medium to large sweet potatoes, diced into small cubes

- 2 cloves garlic, minced

- 1 tablespoon toasted sesame oil (or olive oil)

- Salt and pepper

r the mango coconut rice:

- 2 teaspoons unrefined coconut oil

- 1 cup unsweetened coconut milk or almond coconut milk (from the carton)

- 1 cup water

- 1 cup uncooked brown rice

- 1 large ripe mango, diced

r the almond butter dressing:

- 1/4 cup natural creamy almond butter

- 3-4 tablespoons fresh orange juice, to thin

- 2 teaspoons pure maple syrup

- 1/2 teaspoon apple cider vinegar

- 1 teaspoon toasted sesame oil (or melted coconut oil or olive oil)

- To garnish: Fresh green onions, cilantro and/or toasted sesame seeds.

INSTRUCTIONS

1. To make the brown rice: Place a medium pot over medium high heat and add in coconut oil and brown rice. Toast rice with the coconut oil for 5 minutes; stirring frequently to toast the rice and infused the coconut oil flavor in.

2. After 5 minutes add in water and coconut milk and bring mixture to a boil, then cover, reduce heat to low and simmer for 45 minutes.

3. After 45 minutes, remove heat, stir with a fork and fluff rice, then recover and let stand for 10 more minutes. Once done, stir in mango and season with a little bit of salt.

4. While the rice is cooking, preheat oven to 375 degrees F. Line a large baking sheet with parchment paper OR generously grease with olive oil. Set aside.

5. Place diced sweet potatoes in a bowl and microwave for 3-4 minutes to help pre-cook them.

6. Place broccoli florets, sweet potato cubes minced garlic on baking sheet. Drizzle sesame oil over the top of the veggies and toss to combine. Bake for 20-30 minutes or until sweet potatoes are tender, stirring veggies & potatoes halfway through.

7. While the veggies roast: make the dressing by whisking together almond butter, orange juice, maple syrup, apple cider vinegar and sesame oil. Taste and adjust as you see fit.

8. To assemble the bowls or do meal prep: Add about 3/4 cup of rice to each bowl/container then top with roasted veggies (distribute evenly) and about 1 1/2 tablespoons of the dressing. Top with green onions, cilantro and toasted sesame seeds, if desired. Serves 4.

NUTRITION

Per serving: 450 calories, 18.5 g fat (3.8 g saturated), 45.7 g carbs, 13.8 g sugar, 14 g fiber, 12.1 g protein

Crunchy Cashew Thai Quinoa Salad

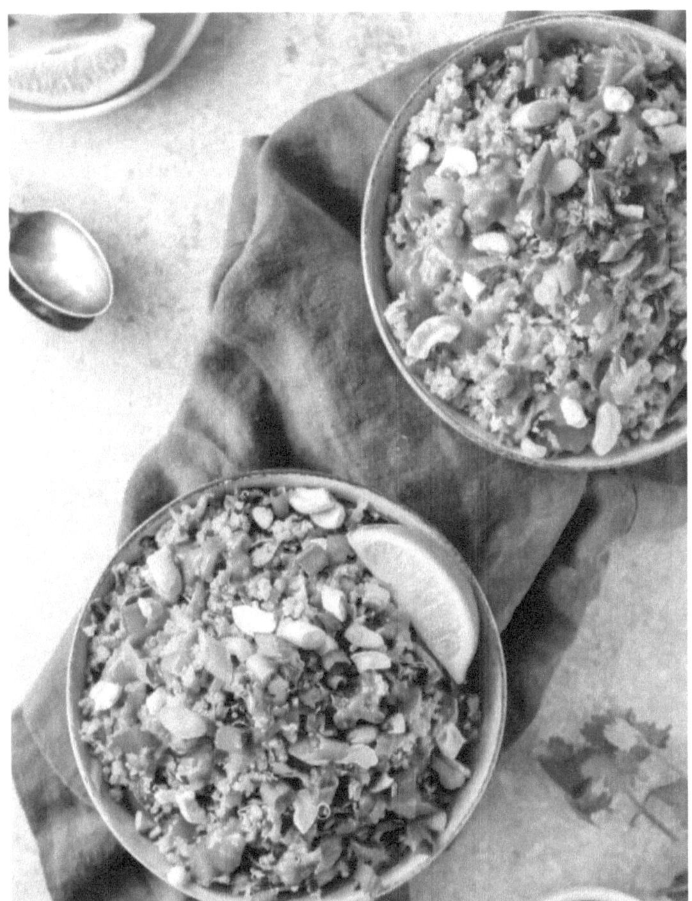

Prep Time: 10 minutes
Cook Time: 15 minutes
Total Time: 25 minutes
Yield: 6

INGREDIENTS

- ¾ cup uncooked quinoa

- 2 cups shredded red cabbage, depending on how much crunch you like

- 1 red bell pepper, diced

- 1/4 cup diced red onion

- 1 cup shredded carrots

- ½ cup chopped cilantro

- ¼ cup diced green onions

- ½ cup cashew halves or peanuts (honey-roasted is good)

- Optional: 1 cup edamame or chickpeas

- Fresh lime, for a bit of tang

r the dressing:

- ¼ cup all natural peanut butter

- 2 teaspoons freshly grated ginger

- 3 tablespoon gluten-free soy sauce or coconut aminos

- 1 tablespoon honey (use agave or pure maple syrup if vegan)

- 1 tablespoon rice vinegar or red wine vinegar

- 1 teaspoon sesame oil

- 1 teaspoon olive oil or more sesame oil

- Water to thin, if necessary

INSTRUCTIONS

1. To cook quinoa: In a medium saucepan, bring 1 ½ cups of water to a boil. Add in quinoa and bring mixture to a boil. Cover, reduce heat to low and let simmer for 15 minutes or until quinoa has absorbed all of the water. Remove from heat and fluff quinoa with fork; place in large bowl and set aside to cool for about 10 minutes. You should have a little over 2 cups of quinoa.

2. To make dressing: Add peanut butter and honey or agave to a medium microwave safe bowl; heat in microwave for 20 seconds. Add in ginger, soy sauce, vinegar, and both sesame and olive oil and stir until mixture is smooth and creamy. If you want a thinner dressing, simply stir in a teaspoon or two of water or olive oil.

3. Add as much or as little dressing as you'd like to the quinoa. I always start out with a little bit of dressing and usually add more to suit my taste preferences. Alternatively you can save the dressing for later and add when you are ready to eat; however the flavors of the dressing usually soak into the salad so I love adding it to the quinoa first.

4. Next fold in red pepper, onion, cabbage, carrots, and cilantro into the quinoa. Garnish with cashews and green onions. Serve chilled or at room temperature with lime wedges, if desired.

NUTRITION

Per serving: 260 calories, 13.5 g fat, 27.7g carbs, 7 g sugar, 4.3 g fiber, 8.6 g protein

Roasted Sweet Potato & Black Bean Salad

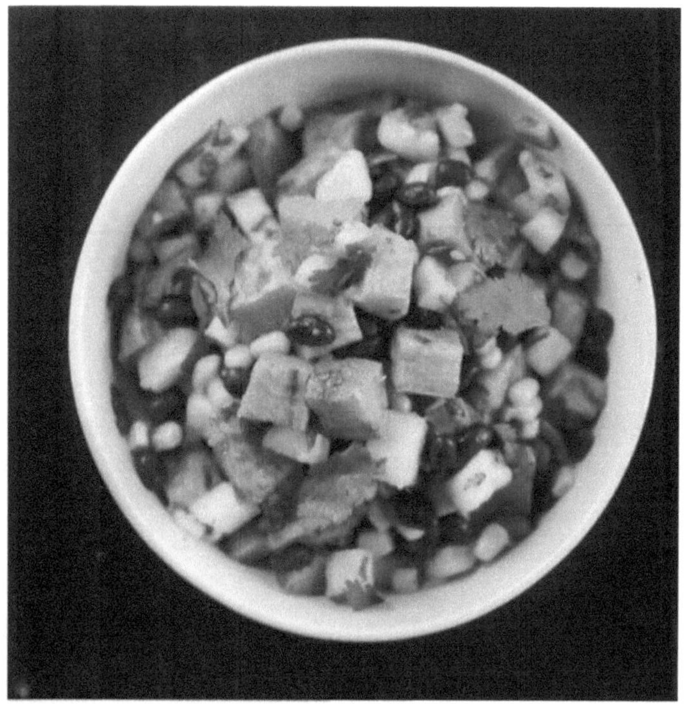

Prep Time: 15 minutes
Cook Time: 30 minutes
Total Time: 45 minutes
Yield: 4

INGREDIENTS

- 1 1/2 pounds sweet potatoes (about 4 medium), cut into 1 inch chunks

- 2 tablespoon olive oil

- 1 tablespoon fresh lime juice

- 1 tablespoon pure maple syrup

- 2 garlic cloves, minced

- 1/2 teaspoon chili powder

- Freshly ground salt and pepper, to taste

- 1 (15 oz) can black beans, rinsed, drained and patted dry

r the salsa:

- 1 cup fresh diced pineapple

- 3/4 cup sweet corn, preferably organic (canned is fine)

- 1/4 cup diecd red onion

- 1 jalapeño, seeded and diced

- 1/3 cup finely chopped fresh cilantro

- salt, to taste

INSTRUCTIONS

1. Preheat oven to 400 degrees F. Add sweet potato cubes to a large bowl.

2. In a small bowl, whisk together olive oil, lime juice maple syrup, garlic and chili powder. Pour over sweet potatoes and toss evenly to distribute.

3. Pour on a baking sheet and spread out evenly. Roast in oven for 25-35 minutes, flipping halfway through, until sweet potatoes are almost fork tender.

4. Remove from oven, cool for a few minutes then immediately transfer to a large bowl or a serving platter. Toss sweet potatoes with black beans and top with salsa!

5. While the sweet potatoes are roasting, make the salsa: In a large bowl, toss pineapple, corn, red onion, jalapeño, cilantro and salt together. Serve warm or cold! Salad can be made a day ahead of time. Serves 4.

NUTRITION

Per serving: 346 calories, 4.6 g fat, 67.7 g carbs, 17.8 g sugar, 11.4 g fiber, 10.5 g protein

Vegan Curried Broccoli Chickpea Salad

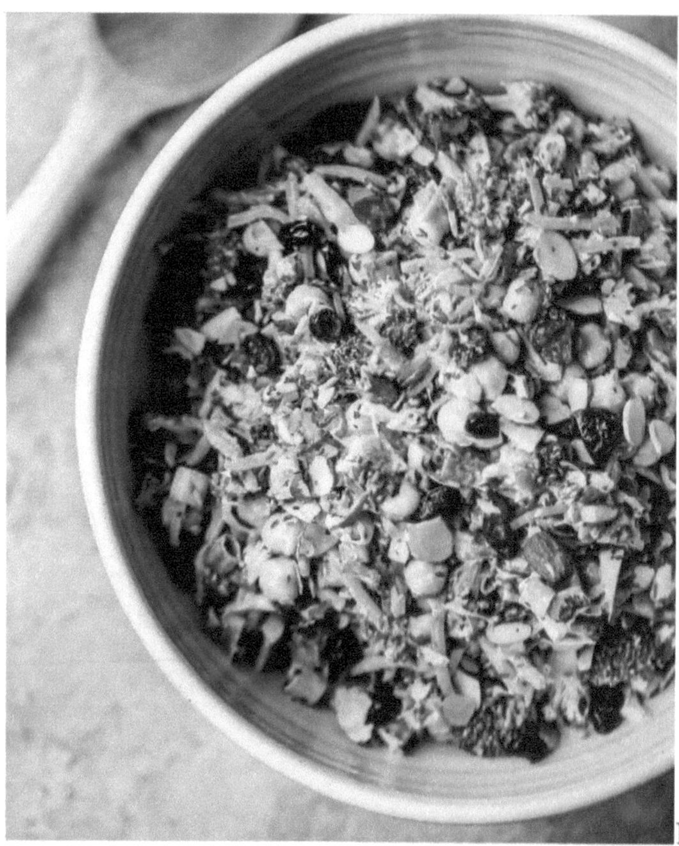

Prep Time: 20 minutes

Total Time: 20 minutes
Yield: 4

INGREDIENTS

For the salad:

- 1 head of broccoli, very finely chopped

- 1 cup shredded carrots

- 1 (15 ounce) can chickpeas, rinsed and drained

- 1/2 cup toasted sliced almonds (can also use chopped roasted almonds)

- 1/2 cup dried cranberries

- 1 bunch green onions, chopped

- ¾ cup chopped fresh cilantro

For the dressing:

- 1/4 cup tahini

- 1/2 large lemon, juiced

- 3-5 tablespoons warm water, to thin dressing

- 1 clove garlic, finely minced

- 1-2 teaspoons pure maple syrup, to sweeten

- 1 teaspoon yellow curry powder

- ½ tablespoon freshly grated ginger

- ½ teaspoon ground turmeric

- ½ teaspoon salt

- Freshly ground black pepper

INSTRUCTIONS

1. In a large bowl, add finely chopped broccoli, chickpeas, carrot, cranberries, green onion, and cilantro. Set aside.

2. Make the dressing by whisking together the following ingredients in a small bowl: tahini, lemon juice, water, garlic, maple syrup, curry powder, ginger, turmeric, salt and pepper. Immediately drizzle over salad and toss to combine. Sprinkle almonds on top and toss a few more times.

3. Serve immediately with fresh squeeze of lemon or place in the fridge for later. Salad will keep well up to 5 days.

• DIY appeal: Unlike many hydroponic systems, deep water culture systems can be made cheaply and easily at home, with a quick run to your pet store and local nursery to pick up the air pump and nutrients.

NUTRITION

Per serving: 434 calories, 17.7 g fat, 56.4 g carbs, 15.6 g sugar, 14.9 g fiber, 15.8 g protein

Tempeh Taco Salad

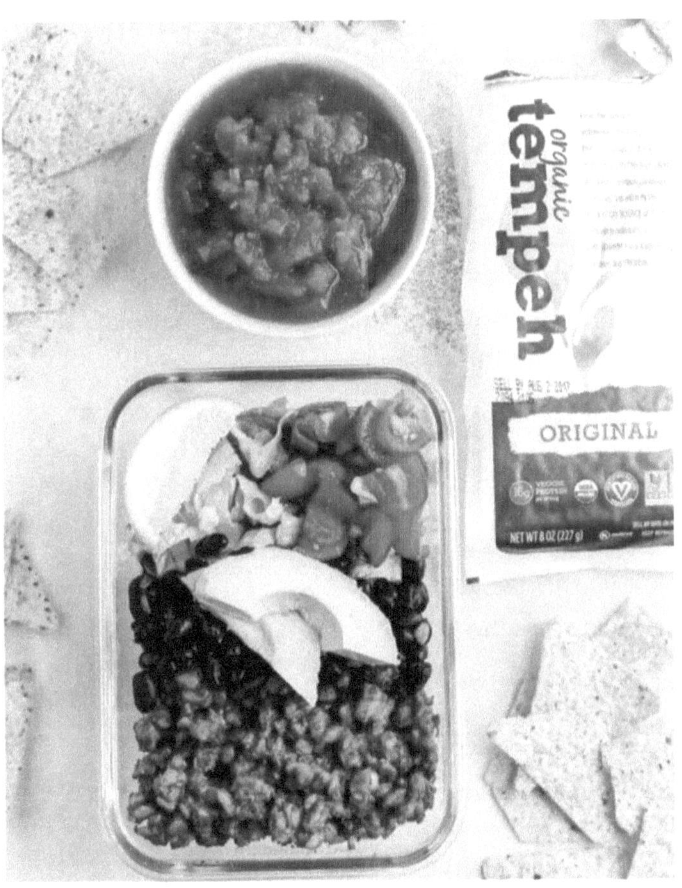

Prep Time: 10 minutes

Cook Time: 10 minutes

Total Time: 20 minutes

Yield: 3 bowls

INGREDIENTS

TEMPEH TACO MEAT

- 8 oz package of Lightlife tempeh (any variety)

- 1 Tablespoon olive or avocado oil

- 1 1/2 Tablespoon chili powder

- 1/2 teaspoon onion powder, garlic powder, paprika, oregano, crushed red pepper, salt and pepper

- 1/4 cup canned tomato sauce

- 1 Tablespoon water

MEAL PREP BOWLS

- 6 cups chopped romaine lettuce

- 1 cup cherry tomatoes, diced

- 1/4 cup red onion, chopped

- 2 Tablespoons fresh cilantro, chopped

- 1/4 teaspoon sea salt

- 3/4 cup cooked black beans

- 1 lime, segmented into three pieces
- 1 avocado, sliced
- fresh salsa, hot sauce and tortilla chips for serving

INSTRUCTIONS

1. Take tempeh out of the package and use your hands to crumble it into a bowl. Heat oil over medium-high heat in a large skillet. Once hot add crumbled tempeh and cook for 3-4 minutes. Add spices, tomato sauce and water into the skillet and toss to combine. Cook for another 3-4 minutes or until most of the liquid has been absorbed. Remove tempeh from stove and let cool.

2. While tempeh is cooking toss together the tomatoes, red onion, cilantro and sea salt in a small bowl.

3. Grab three meal prep containers and add the following ingredients to each: 2 cups romaine lettuce, 1/3 of the tomato and onion mixture, 1/2 cup tempeh, 1/4 cup black beans, one lime slice. You can add the avocado at this time, but it will likely turn brown so I recommend adding it right before you enjoy the bowl.

4. Serve salad bowls with fresh salsa and hot sauce as the dressing and tortillas chips on the side.

NUTRITION

Per serving: 363 calories, 16 g fat, 36 g carbs, 7 g sugar, 21 g fiber, 23 g protein

One-Pot Black Bean Soup

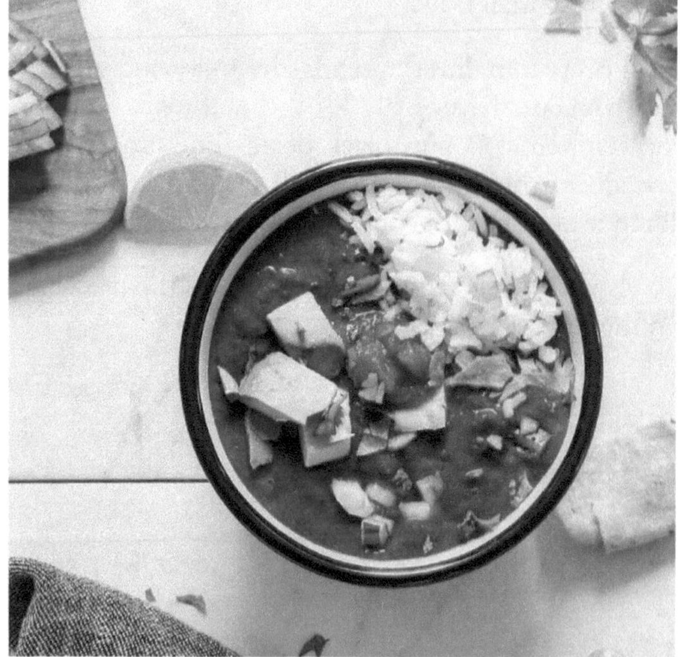

Prep Time: 5 minutes

Cook Time: 25 minutes

Total Time: 30 minutes

Yield: 4

INGREDIENTS

SOUP

- 1 Tbsp oil (or sub water)
- 1 cup diced white or yellow onion
- 3 cloves garlic (minced)
- 1/4 tsp each sea salt + black pepper (more to taste // depends on saltiness of broth)
- 2 15-ounce cans black beans* (slightly drained)
- 2 cups vegetable broth (or store bought)
- 2 tsp ground cumin (for smokiness)
- 1 ½ tsp chili powder
- 1/4 tsp ground coriander
- 1-2 chipotle peppers in adobo sauce (optional // for heat)
- 3 Tbsp chopped vegan dark chocolate (for depth of flavor // we like Theo Dark Chocolate Sea Salt // or sub with 1 Tbsp cacao powder)

FOR SERVING optional

- Lime
- Avocado
- Cilantro
- Onion

- Hot sauce
- Salsa

INSTRUCTIONS

1. Heat a large pot over medium heat. Once hot, add oil (or water), onion, and garlic. Season with a pinch each salt and pepper and sauté for 4-5 minutes.
   2. Add black beans, vegetable broth, cumin, chili powder, coriander, chipotle peppers (optional – start with the lesser amount and work up // adjust to preferred heat level), dark chocolate, and remaining salt and pepper (a couple healthy pinches each).
   3. Bring back to a simmer over medium heat, then reduce heat to low and cook uncovered for about 15-20 minutes (the longer it simmers, the more the flavors develop).
   4. Taste and adjust flavor as needed, adding chipotle peppers for spice, chocolate for depth of flavor, cumin or chili powder for smokiness, or more salt and pepper to taste.
   5. Enjoy as is, or pair with cooked grains such as rice or quinoa. Topping options include fresh lime, avocado or guacamole, cilantro, onion, hot sauce, and/or salsa!
   6. Store soup well covered in the refrigerator up to 5-7 days. Will keep in the freezer for 1 month (oftentimes longer).

NUTRITION

Per serving: 242 calories, 7 g fat (2 g saturated), 37.4 g carbs, 4.1 g sugar, 660 mg sodium, 13.1 g fiber, 10.6 g protein

Roasted Rainbow Vegetable Bowl

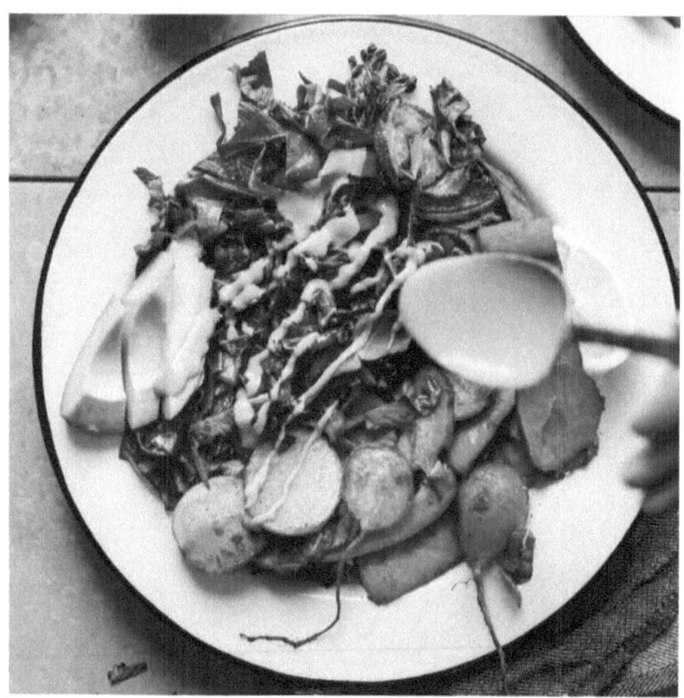

Prep Time: 5 minutes
Cook Time: 25 minutes
Total Time: 30 minutes
Yield: 2

INGREDIENTS

VEGETABLES

- 3-4 medium red or yellow baby potatoes (sliced into 1/4-inch rounds)
- 1/2 large sweet potato (skin on // sliced into 1/4-inch rounds)
- 2 large carrots (halved and sliced)
- 1 medium beet (sliced)
- 4 medium radishes (halved)

- 2 Tbsp avocado or melted coconut oil (divided // if oil-free, sub water or vegetable broth)
- 1 tsp curry powder (divided)
- 1/2 tsp sea salt (divided)
- 1 cup cabbage (thinly sliced)
- 1 medium red pepper (thinly sliced)
- 1 cup broccolini (roughly chopped)
- 2 cups chopped collard greens or kale (organic when possible)

TOPPINGS

- 1 medium lemon (juiced // ~3 Tbsp or 45 ml as original recipe is written // divided)
- 2 Tbsp tahini (divided)
- 2 Tbsp hemp seeds (divided)
- 1/2 medium avocado (divided // optional)

INSTRUCTIONS

1. Preheat oven to 400 degrees F (204 C) and line two baking sheets with parchment paper (or more baking sheets if increasing batch size).

2. To one baking sheet, add the potatoes, sweet potatoes, carrots, beets, and radishes and drizzle with half of the oil (or water), curry powder, and sea salt (as original recipe is written- 1 Tbsp (15 ml) oil (or water), 1/2 tsp curry powder, and 1/4 tsp sea salt). Toss to combine. Bake for a total of 20-25 minutes or until golden brown and tender.

3. To the second baking sheet, add the cabbage, bell pepper, and broccolini. Drizzle with with the remaining half of the oil (or water), curry powder, and sea salt (as original recipe is written- 1 Tbsp (15 ml) oil (or water), 1/2 tsp curry powder, and 1/4 tsp sea salt). Toss to combine.

4. When the potatoes/carrots hit the 10-minute mark, add the second pan to the oven and bake for a total of 15-20 minutes.

In the last 5 minutes of baking, add the collard greens or kale to either pan and roast until tender and bright green.

5. To serve, divide vegetables between serving plates and garnish with avocado (optional) and season with lemon juice, tahini, hemp seeds, and another pinch of sea salt (optional). You could also garnish with any fresh herbs you have!

6. Best when fresh. Store leftovers covered in the refrigerator for 3-4 days. Reheat in a 350-degree F (176 C) oven or on the stovetop over medium heat until hot.

NUTRITION

Per serving: 519 calories, 14.5 g fat, 59.2 g carbs, 13.7 g sugar, 518 mg sodium, 12.5 g fiber, 13.2 g protein